About These

These booklets were developed by Narinder Kapur, consultant neuropsychologist and Head of Neuropsychology in Cambridge, England. They were based on earlier booklets and materials in previous posts. While in Cambridge, he won awards for his clinical and academic work, and for his management suggestions.

Narinder Kapur is currently visiting Professor of Neuropsychology at University College London and honorary consultant neuropsychologist at Imperial College NHS Trust. He is Past-President of the British Neuropsychological Society, and was awarded a Lifetime Achievement Award by the British Psychological Society.

These rehabilitation booklets can be purchased –

In **electronic** form for Kindle – by buying on Amazon

In **electronic** form for iBooks – by buying in iTunes. In the UK, the web address is – www.apple.com/uk/ibooks/

In **electronic** form at – www.rehab-booklets.com

In **print** form – by buying on Amazon

The *Cambridge Memory Manual*, which deals with improving everyday memory, can be purchased separately –

In **electronic** form for Kindle – by buying on Amazon

In **electronic** form for iBooks – by buying in iTunes. In the UK, the web address is – www.apple.com/uk/ibooks/

In **electronic** form – at www.cambridgememorymanual.com

In **print** form – by buying on Amazon

Any surplus proceeds from sales of these booklets go towards supporting Neuropsychology in India and to the Arpana Charity Hospital, Karnal, Haryana, northern India

© Narinder Kapur, 2017

[2]

Contents (pages numbers are bottom centre in book)

1. Coping with Anger 4

2. Concentration Tips... 8

3. Managing Stress... 12

4. Handling Fatigue 20

5. Getting a Good Night's Sleep.................................... 28

6. Going Back to Work after a Brain Injury 32

7. Study Tips for Students 36

8. Caring for a Confused Patient................................... 44

9. Improving Word-Finding Ability............................... 56

10. Advice for Staff Caring for Disturbed Patients 60

COPING WITH ANGER

What is anger?

Anger is a response that may range from mild irritation to intense rage. Although being angry can sometimes help motivate you to create change for the better, problems in controlling anger can adversely affect your health, your work, your home life, and the wellbeing of others – so it is important to deal with it well. There is nothing wrong with occasionally being angry, as it is natural and normal to feel upset in some situations. However, it is important that you avoid becoming angry to an extreme degree or too often, or to the extent that it affects your wellbeing and that of others.

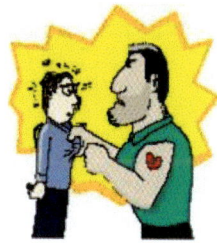

Getting angry usually consists of three things – thinking negatively about something that has happened – often as an automatic reaction, experiencing unpleasant feelings, and saying/doing things which directly result from your feeling upset. You may be verbally or physically aggressive to others, you may sulk and refuse to interact with others, and you may neglect to look after yourself properly. It can result in depression, low self-esteem, alcohol / drug abuse and high blood pressure.

What makes people angry?

There are **four** main types of situations that make people angry -

1. **Frustrations.** These include not being able to get something you want or not being able to do something as well as you want to do it – e.g. losing your way when you are trying to go somewhere, misplacing something at home or work, not being able to watch your favourite TV programme, missing an important phone call, failing an important exam, or not being able to do things by yourself that you once could do easily.

2. **Personal discomfort or loss.** These could be things that cause you discomfort or distress, such as getting wet in the rain, spilling a drink over your clothes, having a physical disability, falling sick, or not getting a good night's sleep. It could also cover money problems, not being able to drive a car, having to move house, losing a job, etc.

3. **Things which other people do.** For example, a neighbour may do something annoying such as playing music too loudly, another car driver could do something to upset you, or someone could ignore you or treat you as inferior.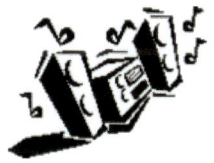

4. **Things which other people say.** Someone may call you names, they may criticise a mistake you have made, interrupt you when you are talking, etc.

Realizing why you may start to get angry

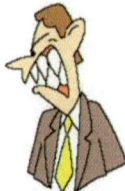
You may not always be aware when you get angry, so ask others around you to let you know. Although you may occasionally appear to get angry for no apparent reason, there are usually some clues that indicate that you may get angry – 'bad day blues', triggers and warning signs. *'Bad day blues'* simply means that you may just be having an off day – you may be tired, perhaps due to lack of sleep; you may have a headache or be in pain; there may be too many people around; or you may just be feeling low. *Triggers* are things which get you going, and usually fall into one of the types mentioned above – frustrations, personal discomfort/loss, things that people do or things that people say. Often we will get angry as a result of several unpleasant things happening together at the same time – e.g. you may be tired after a poor night's sleep, get wet in the rain, slip and hurt yourself, miss a bus, arrive late for an important meeting, and then be criticised for being late. *Warning signs* may be your heart thumping, feeling tense in your body, raising the tone of your voice, speaking faster, feeling restless or feeling hot.

Being more aware of these factors, and the thoughts that go through your head, will help you understand better why you get angry and help you deal more effectively with the situation.

Coping better with anger situations

Try to see an angry situation as a challenge, and as a chance to try out some of the techniques below. There are **seven** main things you can do to help you cope better with anger -

1. Avoid trigger situations in the first place / be prepared

If you have kept a record of what happens when you get angry, this may help you to find a pattern - for example times, places, people, etc, that are likely to make you angry. It may be worth either avoiding such situations in the first place or dealing with the specific triggers or anger behaviour in particular ways. On the basis of how you have become angry in the past, try to anticipate situations that may give rise to feelings of anger. This allows you to prepare for them. By anticipating the situation you have time to plan and rehearse what you will do and say. If possible, remove yourself from the situation before you reach 'boiling point'. Have a place to go or something to do that will distract and relax you. If becoming angry is secondary to frustrations at not being able to do things like before, you may find you have to reduce your expectations.

2. Think about people differently

Since we often get angry as a result of what people say or do, it is natural to concentrate on people's faults. Try to think of the good qualities that the person has and the helpful things they have done in the past. Try to see things from their angle. In addition, avoid taking any remarks or actions as a personal attack on you – it is possible that the person behaves like that with other people as well. Be more forgiving of others.

3. Think about events differently

If you sense you are about to get angry about something, pause and think twice about the situation. Have you got all the facts, and are the facts right? Have you simply 'got the wrong end of the stick'? Ask yourself which of the four types of anger this is, mentioned on page 1 of the booklet. Events are seldom as important or as awful as they first seem. Practise giving the event a mark out of 20 – firstly, out of 10 for how important it is, and then out of 10 for how awful it is. Even if an event is very upsetting, the chances are that you can deal with the consequences, and it is worth keeping this in mind by saying – '*I can handle this*'.

How you see a situation often affects whether it makes you angry or not. Therefore, it's not so much what happens that's important – it's how you take it, and how you think about it later on. Just as some people may see a heavy snowfall as unpleasant while others may see it as beautiful, some people may see an event as stressful while others may see it as a blessing in disguise. Replace thoughts such as 'its terrible and everything is ruined' with 'it may be frustrating and a reason to be upset, but it's not the end of the world'. If you find yourself becoming 'stressed out' over an event, say to yourself things such as – '*relax, it's not so important, it's not so awful*' OR '*what's the worst thing that could happen here – I can deal with it*'.

Making a joke about a stressful situation can also help you see something in perspective and prevent feelings of anger.

4. Manage your feelings better

Try not to keep your feelings bottled up inside you. Always try to put your feelings into words – tell others politely how you feel. Some people find that saying calming things to themselves helps (e.g. '*relax*', '*take it easy*'), or saying positive things like, '*This is a test of my resilience and my coping skills*'. Others find that it helps to try slow, regular breathing for a short while, counting 1-2-3 when breathing in, and when breathing out saying a calming word. Find out if any of these techniques works for you, and if so, remember to use it when you get angry.

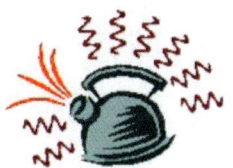

5. Say things differently

Often, your immediate reaction in an angry situation is not the best one, and that applies particularly to what you say – whether this is swearing, calling someone names, belittling yourself, etc. Try to stay 'semi-detached' from the situation. Don't say the first thing that comes into your head - think before you speak. Avoid shouting or swearing. If you do end up saying something, try to stay calm and speak slowly. Use 'polite' words or phrases, such as '*please*', '*would you mind*', etc. Start any negative comment with '*I appreciate, I sympathise, but....*' Try to make general rather than personal comments – e.g. instead of '*you sometimes treat me like a child*', say '*people sometimes treat me like a child*'. Avoid using words such as '*always*', '*never*', '*very*', '*ought*', '*should*', or '*must*' when talking about yourself or others in heated situations. Rather, use words such as '*sometimes*', '*a little*' and '*perhaps*'.

[6]

6. Do things differently

Try not to react immediately in an angry situation. Pause for a few moments and see if there are any other ways of responding. If you suffer a loss or personal discomfort, e.g. if you spoil a piece of clothing or lose a credit card, try and find a way of solving the problem – could you wear something else or borrow cash till the credit card is replaced? If someone annoys you by what they are doing, is it possible simply to ignore them, speak to them politely, or ask someone else to intervene? If you are frustrated that you cannot find something, even after retracing your steps and looking in all the likely places, just leave the situation and come back after half an hour, or ask someone to help you find it. If you are in an argument with someone, it may also help here to leave the situation completely – go for a walk, do physical exercise / sports, make a cup of tea, suck a sweet, chew some gum, or listen to some music – and then come back to the situation later. There may often be a simple solution to the situation which will become apparent when you are in a calmer state of mind. If you still feel very angry, talk to a friend or family member you trust, or to a healthcare professional.

7. Try some exercises
These exercises may help you to think and behave differently in anger situations.
(a) **Play positive.** Think of an unpleasant event. Then try and think of something good or positive about that event. For example, a downpour where you got soaked and your clothes ruined…..could mean you can buy a new set of clothes!
(b) **Generate ambiguous situations.** Think of situations that could make you angry but where there could be other explanations. For example, a man jumping a queue at the supermarket till. He could be rude, but he could also have an urgent medical appointment or could be a policeman having to attend an accident.
(c) **Put yourself in their shoes.** Imagine making a critical remark about someone. Then pretend he / she did the same to you. How would you feel? Think of other examples.

Regularly read this booklet
If you have had an anger outburst, it is a good idea to read this booklet soon afterwards, to help you see where you went wrong, and how you might do better next time. It may be useful to set aside a regular time each week to read this booklet, and to apply some of the ideas to events that have happened to you in the past week. Note things you did right, and things you may have done wrong. Try to see each time you became angry as a learning experience – so that you realise ways of reacting that you should avoid in the future. Remember also to note the parts you did well – ways that you found particularly useful in dealing with a situation. On those occasions when you successfully managed a stressful event, give yourself a 'pat on the back'.

Carers – If you are a friend or family member of someone with anger outbursts, stay calm, listen to them in a sympathetic way, allow them time and space to express their emotions and set boundaries for what is acceptable and unacceptable behaviour.

The advice in this leaflet is not a substitute for treatment. Seek professional help if you or others remain concerned about your anger coping skills.
Other helpful resources can be found at – www.mind.org.uk

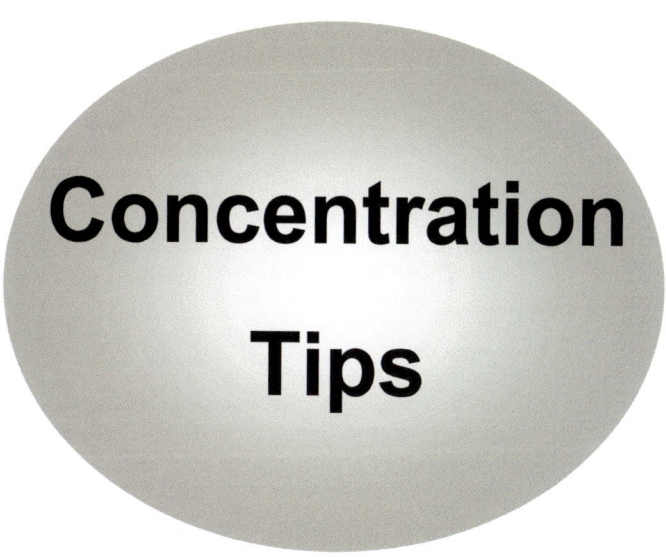

Concentration Tips

Be motivated

- We concentrate better on something if we are motivated to do it and enjoy doing it. Try to see an enjoyable side to the activity you are doing, and try to link it in to goals/aims that you hold dear.

Be well organized

- Try to be organized into a routine, so that you do set things at set times of the day, and set things on set days of the week.
- Try to be organized where you live and work - have set places where you put things, have these places labelled if possible, always put things away after you use them, etc.

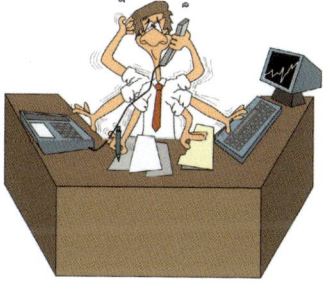

Don't overload yourself

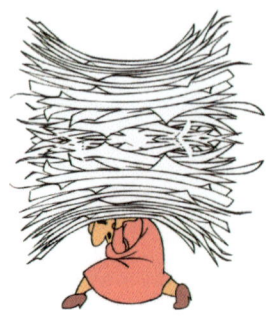

- Don't overload yourself with too many things to do - do one thing at a time.

- Break a big job into smaller, easily achievable parts. Write these down on a piece of note-paper, or on a white board, with times for each activity. Set yourself a goal of finishing each part at a set time, and then move on to the next part. Do not leave something half-done.

- Don't rush tasks – take your time, and pace yourself.

- Have regular breaks. If you are sitting down for a while, stretch your legs and walk around. If you eyes have been focused on close-up material, look out of a window for a while.

- Know your good times, and good days. Do difficult tasks when you are feeling relaxed and fresh. Keep simple tasks for when you are tired or not feeling so good.

Check carefully

- If you are doing something that involves different activities in sequence, such as cooking a meal, make up a check-list of things to do, put it in a prominent place, and tick off each thing after you do it.

- Allow for the possibility that you may run out of time, or that things may not go according to plan. Don't panic if things go wrong.

- From time to time, make sure that everything is going to plan.

- If you are doing a task where you might easily make mistakes – such as checking figures in a bank account – double-check your answers, or get someone else to check them.

Stay on track

- If you find your concentration wanders from one minute to the next, use a watch timer or a kitchen timer that goes off every 10 mins to remind you to keep on track. Gradually increase the time before any alarm goes off. Watches or other devices that vibrate at set intervals can also be used as ways to cue you to stay on track.

- If your mind is often wandering when doing something, put up a little sign in front of you – KEEP ON TRACK – or repeat this phrase to yourself every now and again.

- If you find your eyes wandering when talking to someone, try to maintain eye-contact by focusing on their eyes. If your mind wanders in a conversation, try asking yourself questions about what is being said, or try to link it to something you find interesting. If someone is speaking too fast, ask them to slow down or repeat what they have said.

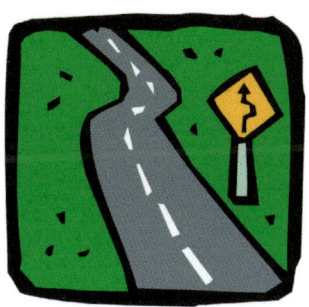

- If you have difficulty concentrating when reading, asking questions and making notes at the time that you read may help you to concentrate better. If you are reading a novel, you could make brief notes on a bookmark, perhaps one with Post-It tape stuck on. If you are reading as part of a course, you could summarise key points on an index card, and keep these cards for future reference. Try to link what you are reading to something interesting or meaningful to you.

Avoid distractions

- Choose the environment that suits you best. Usually a quiet setting with no distractions (e.g. TV or people talking) is better for concentrating on an activity, such as reading. If you find that ear plugs/headphones help, then use them. If you are in a room at home, have a DO NOT DISTURB sign on the door. Remove any clutter from your desk. Avoid working near a window, as there may be distractions from outside. If you work better when together with others who are also working, such as in a library, then work there. If your mind wanders during a lecture, sitting in the front is usually better for concentration.

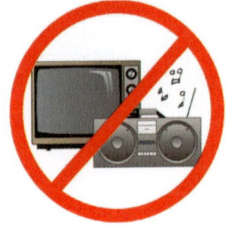

- If you concentrate better when someone else is doing a similar thing, try to discuss your work with him/her, and do it jointly if possible.

- Some people find that playing board games or computer games helps their concentration. While this may not apply to everyone, there is no harm in trying this, if only to boost your self-confidence for being able to concentrate over a period of time. Start off with shorter/simpler games, and then move on to longer/more complicated ones.

Take it easy

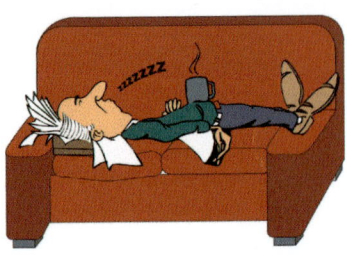

- If you are anxious about something and it is affecting your concentration, try to deal with it. Use any relaxation techniques you have learned. If it is constantly on your mind, divert your mind onto other things or do something more relaxing, such as listening to music.

- If your concentration lets you down or you do something badly, try to stay calm. Figure out what you did wrong, and decide how you can do better next time. Be Patient - Be Positive – Persevere ('P-P-P').

- If you do well, tell yourself this, and give yourself a little treat. This will help you realise that you are getting better, and will help to improve your self-confidence.

- Try to take part in sports and recreational activities, especially those that involve being with other people. Remember to use family members, close friends, psychologists, etc to help you out if you get into real difficulties.

The advice in this leaflet should be considered in the context of your own particular circumstances and any other support or advice that you receive

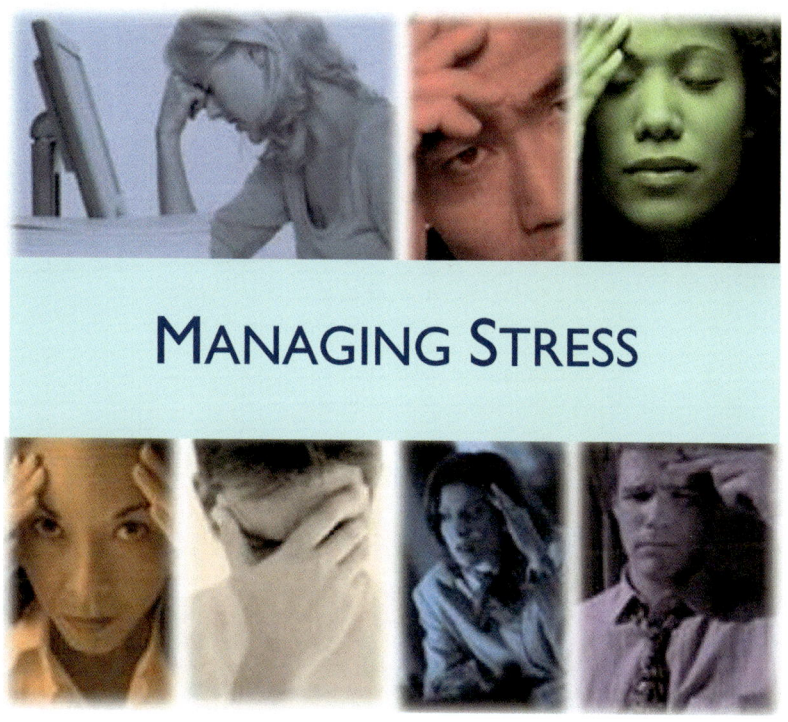

Managing Stress

WHAT IS STRESS?

Stress is very common and is experienced by many people. There are many different factors which can help to make a person feel stressed. These can vary from person to person. However, common factors include demands from work or family, money problems, health problems and difficulties getting on with others.

Recognising stress

It is important to recognise the symptoms of stress. Common signs include:
- Feeling overwhelmed
- Heart thumping or beating faster
- Difficulty sleeping
- Feeling wound up and tense
- Losing your temper with those around you
- Weight loss or weight gain
- Drinking too much alcohol
- Feeling tired much of the time

The impact of stress

Stress can have a negative impact upon your physical and mental health if it is not managed properly. It can disturb your sleep, affect your mood and stop you concentrating.

The impact of stress can also affect how well you get on with other people and stop you functioning effectively with others.

You can't completely avoid stress since it is a natural part of everyday life, and in some circumstances a certain amount of stress can be helpful to keep you motivated. So, for example, if you have a deadline at work you might experience some level of stress which then ensures that you work towards meeting your target. However, when stress becomes overwhelming and prevents you from functioning effectively it is unhelpful. It is therefore important that you find ways to manage stress which help you to keep mentally and physically healthy.

[13]

Managing Stress

MANAGING STRESS

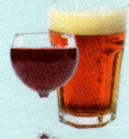

Most people try to manage stress on their own. However, while some ways of coping seem to work initially, they may actually be unhelpful or harmful in the longer term. Examples of potentially damaging ways of coping include smoking, drinking too much alcohol, overeating, opting out by watching excessive amounts of television, and taking drugs.

There are many healthy ways to cope with stress, some of which are described below. Everyone is different and you may wish to try out a number of the ideas in this booklet to discover which ones work best for you. If you are aware that you are already trying to manage your stress in an unhealthy way, try to replace it with a more healthy strategy.

Dealing with stress in a positive way
The first step in learning to manage your stress is to become more aware of which factors trigger stress. You may already be aware of certain factors, but there may be others which are less obvious. You could keep a diary which records when you are feeling stressed. This should help you identify which situations you find most difficult and will help you think about which parts of your life you could consider changing.

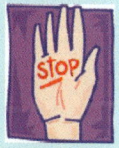

The next step is to look at whether there are things you can do to deal directly with the factors in your life which make you feel stressed. This could include some of the following –

- Learning to say no to others when you know that you do not have the time or the knowledge / experience to do what they ask is a very important skill. It can feel difficult to begin with, especially if you are the type of person who likes to be helpful. However, it should get easier with practice.

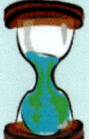

- Ensure that you give yourself plenty of time to do what you need to do. It is very stressful to rush from one activity to the next, allowing extra time will help to take the pressure off.

[14]

3

Managing Stress

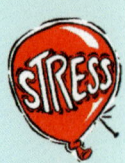

- Find out whether there are particular people that make you feel more stressed, and if it is possible, try and reduce your interactions with them.

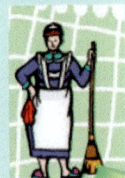

- Take a good look at your life and think about whether there is anything that you could change which could make things easier. This could include looking at changing your job, reducing your hours at work, or getting help in the house.

If you are overwhelmed by a situation and you are unable to see it in another way, it can be useful to talk things over with a trusted relative or friend. It is possible that they may be able to look at the situation differently and bring another point of view. Try and remember that we all need help from time to time, and sharing our difficulties with others can be extremely helpful. It can also be helpful to remind yourself that while life may feel difficult at the moment, in time the situation may improve. Comparing the difficult situation to the worst possible thing that could happen may also you to keep it in perspective. Also, it can be useful to remind yourself that, whilst a situation may feel very difficult now, over time things can improve.

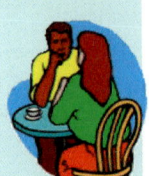

Most people will suffer some stresses which cannot easily be avoided. In these situations, it may be helpful to look at ways of helping you cope in other ways. The following are ideas which could help.

Do something physical
Exercise is a great way of relaxing and can help to counteract stress as well as improving your general physical health. Exercise can lift your mood. It can help you forget the problems of the day and provide space in a busy schedule where you can release tension. The sense of satisfaction you experience after taking exercise can help improve your mood and raise your self esteem, giving you more confidence to deal with the challenges you face.

[15]

Managing Stress

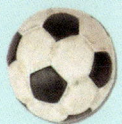

To increase the likelihood that you will continue to exercise regularly it is a good idea to try and pick an activity you enjoy. It can also be a good idea to try and take part in an activity which brings you into contact with others. This could be a team sport such as tennis or football, an exercise class or dancing. This could increase your social life as well as helping you mentally and physically.

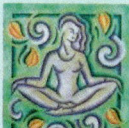

Relaxation exercises can also be a useful way of helping you to wind down. There are two main types of relaxation exercises. One is called *Progressive Muscle Relaxation*. This involves tensing and relaxing your muscles. With practice you will become aware of the physical signs of stress and you can quickly relax your muscles and bring about a state of mental calmness.

Some people who have had physical health problems may find it difficult to tense and relax their muscles and it may be better for them to use a different kind of relaxation called *Guided Imagery*. In this type of relaxation, the goal is to imagine yourself in a peaceful setting. With practice, you will find it easier to quickly imagine yourself into this place. Both types of relaxation exercise are widely available on CD and can be purchased in shops and via websites.

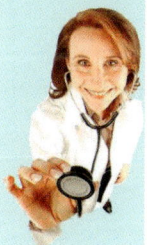

If you have not exercised for some time it is sensible to check with your doctor that it is safe for you to begin exercising.

Manage your time better

If you have many demands on your time and energies it can be useful to write a list of the things which need to be finished and then try and deal first with those which are most important. If possible, you could think of asking others to do certain tasks for you. If you find it difficult to make decisions about which tasks are most important you could discuss it with a trusted friend or colleague.

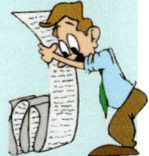

When you have a busy life it can be hard to find time for yourself. However, if you can do this regularly you may feel less stressed and be more effective when you resume your other

[16]

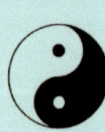

activities. People will vary in terms of how they relax. However, possible ideas include having a warm bath, watching a good film, listening to music or reading a book.

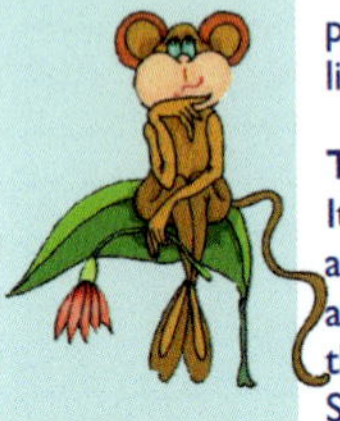

Think differently

It can help to be more aware of your thinking habits, especially any negative ones. Some people may be at risk of suffering stress as a result of the way they think about themselves, how they think of others and the way they look at the world around them. Some thinking styles which can be particularly unhelpful are described below, together with alternative ways of thinking that may be better.

Negative ways of thinking can result in you feeling more stressed at work and at home. By becoming more aware of how you think, you can begin to question some of your automatic thoughts and behaviour.

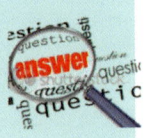

ALL-OR-NOTHING THINKING – This means seeing things in a very narrow way. People who have this style of thinking often make sense of the world by putting people and situations into one of two totally opposite groups – e.g. *you are either with us or against us… either you give me everything or give me nothing.* So things are seen as good or bad, right or wrong ~ **INSTEAD** ~ **try and think** that most situations have some positive and some negative aspects to them. Things are rarely as clear-cut as this style of thinking would suggest. Better ways of thinking are – *it could be a bit of both and that's fine… even if I don't get everything, that'll do for the time being.*

MAGNIFYING THE NEGATIVE – This occurs when something unpleasant about a situation or a person is made much more important and much worse than it is – e.g. *this situation/person is absolutely awful* ~ **INSTEAD** ~ **you might think** – *this is not as important or as terrible as it seems. In a few months time, I'll look back at this as being not so bad.*

MINIMISING THE POSITIVE – This is when something good about a person or situation is played down – e.g. *he/she/it may be good but still not perfect* ~ **INSTEAD** ~ **try and think** – *that's really good and I'm pleased about it.*

[17]

Managing Stress

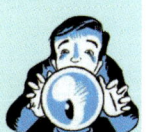

SELECTIVE EVIDENCE – This is when you only take into account one part of the picture and ignore other parts – e.g. only thinking about the mistakes you or others have made in the past, and not the times you/others got it right ~ **INSTEAD** ~ you could try to put events in context and look at the broader picture.

MIND-READING – This means guessing that people are thinking bad things about you, or are trying to cause you stress, when there is no real reason to think this – e.g. *they must think I am stupid… they do this on purpose to upset me* ~ **INSTEAD** ~ **think along the lines of** – *I can't really tell how they think…I can't be sure why they did this, maybe there was a good reason I'm not aware of.*

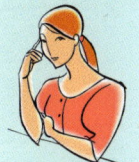

OVER-GENERALISATION – This relates to drawing conclusions from one negative instance and then applying it to other situations. People often use the words 'very' and 'always' to over-generalise about an event or person e.g. *he/she is always late* ~ **INSTEAD** ~ *he/she was late on that occasion, but in general he/she has kept to time.*

PESSIMISTIC PREDICTION – This is when you think you will be unable to cope with the consequences of an event and automatically think that the future looks bleak – e.g. *I don't know how I am going to cope, everything will end up as a disaster* ~ **INSTEAD** ~ *I've handled similar/worse situations in the past, everything will work out OK in the long-run.*

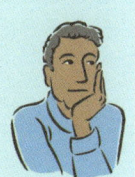

BEING A PERFECTIONIST – If you often use the words *should* or *must* or *ought*, it is possible that you have firm ideas about how you and others are expected to behave. It may also be a sign that you have too high expectations of yourself or others. This can result in a feeling that nothing you or others do is good enough, resulting in you pushing yourself and those around you harder and harder to reach goals which may not be realistic.

[18]

Managing Stress

Finally...
We hope that this booklet will give you some ideas which will help you feel more in control of your life. Some of them may be more helpful than others, give yourself time to try them out to see what best works with you.
However, if after trying to use these strategies you feel things are still getting on top of you, it may be worth going to see your GP.

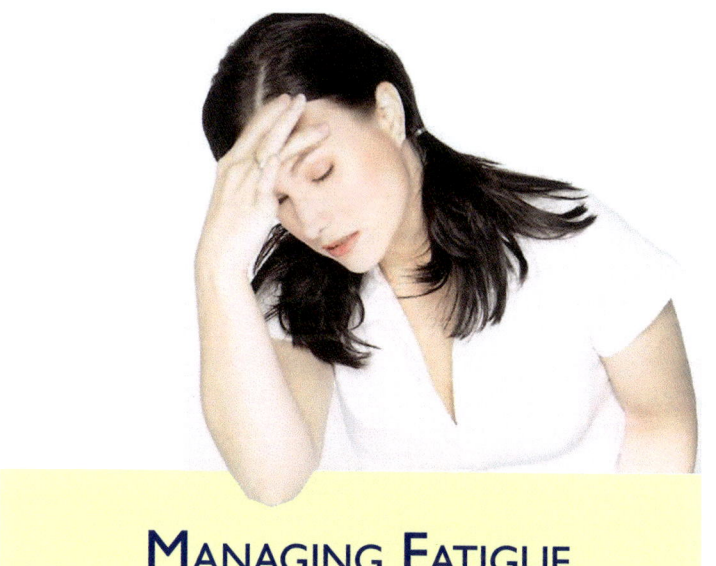

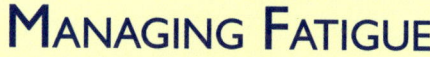

Managing Fatigue

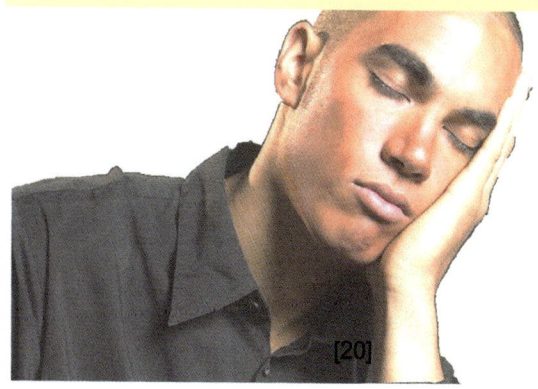

WHAT IS FATIGUE?

Fatigue or tiredness is a natural condition, experienced by everyone at some point. It usually follows either intense physical or mental activity and generally goes away after a period of rest. Physical fatigue can occur after taking exercise whilst mental fatigue can follow long periods of concentration.

Some people experience fatigue even when they have not been very active and this type of tiredness may not disappear after rest. This type of tiredness has been called chronic fatigue. It can be a condition in its own right or it can be due to other factors. These include physical factors such as illness, infection and injury and psychological factors such as depression or anxiety.

While fatigue is different for everyone, common complaints include extreme tiredness, exhaustion, weakness or feeling completely drained of energy. It is a frustrating condition that can result in despair and hopelessness.

This leaflet will help you to understand more about fatigue and suggests coping strategies to improve your quality of life.

What causes fatigue?
Things that trigger fatigue will vary from person to person so it may help to be aware of the things which often trigger your fatigue. Common activities which can trigger mental fatigue include a busy day at work, preparing a meal for lots of people, driving for long distances without a break, trying to follow a conversation in a noisy environment or working at a computer. Activities that can trigger physical fatigue include exercising and doing physically demanding tasks.

How can you recognise fatigue?
It will be helpful to be able to know when you are starting to become tired out. Being aware of early warning signs will mean you can rest before you feel overcome with fatigue. Family, friends or work colleagues may be able to help you notice warning signs. Possible signs may include yawning, heavy limbs, eyes losing focus or drooping, irritability or loss of concentration.

[21]

MANAGING FATIGUE

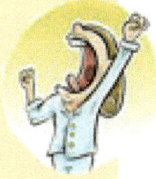

For many people, a sense of extreme tiredness does not go away over time. It is therefore likely to be helpful to think about ways of organising your life so that you can manage the symptoms of fatigue. This can help to give you the best possible quality of life. The following factors are worth keeping in mind –

Emotional factors

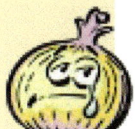

Tiredness can be a symptom of depression. Other common symptoms of depression include having negative thoughts and feeling hopeless about the future. Sometimes when people say that are tired and exhausted they are actually feeling low in mood. If you believe that you may be depressed it could be useful to talk through how you are feeling with a healthcare professional. Treatments for depression included psychological therapy such as cognitive behavioural therapy and antidepressant medication. Some people notice an increase in their energy levels as their depression resolves. When people feel tired and low they tend to say negative things to themselves, and this can make things worse. One way to deal with this is to say positive things to yourself such as –

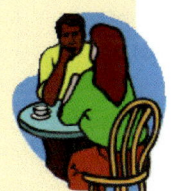

1. I'm feeling tired, but I've felt much more tired before and I've handled that well.
2. I'm feeling tired but if I tell someone he/she will be able to help me out.
3. I'm feeling tired but that doesn't affect my ability to do many of the things I have to do.
4. I'm feeling tired so I'll have a short nap to boost my energy.
5. I'm feeling tired but if I take things slowly I'll be fine in a little while.

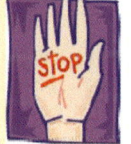

Stress can also affect your energy levels. If you are stressed it can cause you to feel overwhelmed and exhausted. There are many ways to try and reduce the level of stress in your life.

[22]

These include making sure you are realistic about what you can do each day and ensuring that you have enough time to relax and do things that help you relax. This could be having a warm bath, reading a book, listening to music or going for a walk or swim.

Prioritising and Planning
If you have fatigue that lingers throughout the day, it is important that you plan your day to ensure that you have the energy to do what is necessary. It can be helpful to decide which activities are most important and try to ensure you do these activities when you have most energy. For many people this is in the morning, but everyone is different.

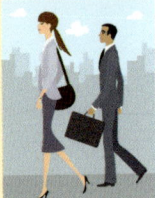

Being aware of what triggers your fatigue can also be helpful as it can allow you to plan your day. For example, before you need to complete an important task, you should try to avoid doing things that usually result in you feeling fatigued.

When you are planning your day, it can be useful to ensure that you have a good mix of activities. For example, you could mix up physical tasks, such as walking to the shops, with less physically demanding activities, such as paying the bills, to make sure that you do not get too physically or mentally exhausted. As you become more aware of which tasks tire you the most, you can plan ahead to make sure you make the best possible use of your energies. For example, if you find doing the supermarket shopping particularly tiring, there are a number of things you could do to minimise this. These could include ordering shopping over the internet, having a rest period before and after shopping, or asking a friend or relative to help you.

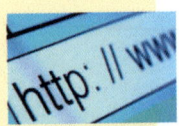

You may also find it helpful to take regular rest breaks during the day. It can be useful to take more frequent, shorter breaks rather than one long rest. You could consider whether you find it better to take a short nap or do something relaxing.

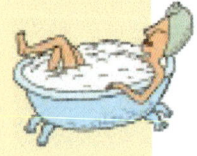

4

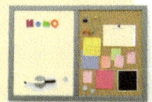

Making Changes to your Work and Home Space

To make the best of your energy, you may wish to design your home and work area to help you manage your daily activities. This could help to lessen the physical and mental effort that is needed to complete an activity. It may be useful to get some extra help around the house, such as hiring a cleaner or a gardener.

It can be helpful to make sure that the things you need regularly are available to hand and organised so you do not waste valuable time and energy looking for them. Try and get into the habit of putting things back in the correct place so you know where they are when you need them again. You may notice that if you do these often enough, they become habits and you do them without thinking about it.

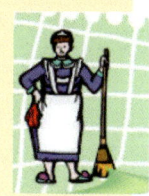

HEALTHY LIVING

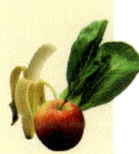

Diet

Eating a healthy and balanced diet is important since some foods can make us feel more lethargic than others. Foods such as sweets, chocolate and cakes which release sugar quickly into the blood may result in you experiencing a quick burst of energy followed by a sharp drop, leaving you feeling fatigued. Foods such as wholemeal bread, pasta fruit and vegetables which release sugar more slowly can help to keep your energy levels over a longer period of time.

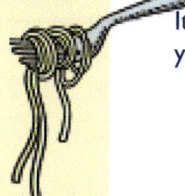

It is therefore important to limit sugary foods whilst ensuring you eat a variety of wholesome foods.

[24]

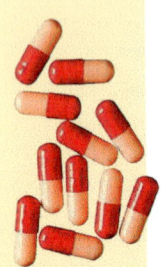

Medication

Some medicines may indirectly help your energy levels. So for example, if depression is adding to your fatigue taking anti-depressants could help improve your mood and increase your energy levels. It is also possible that side-effects from the medication you take could include drowsiness. It is important that you discuss any concerns you may have about your medication with your doctor who will be able to advise you further.

Exercise

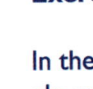

In the long term, doing regular exercise will help your fatigue levels, even though at first you may feel tired after a period of exercise. For some people exercise has been linked to improved mood, better quality of sleep and increased energy levels.

Some professionals suggest trying to do 30 minutes of moderately intense activity five times a week. There are many ways you can try to achieve this e.g. walking rather than taking the bus or car, swimming, going to a local exercise class. Gardening can be a good form of exercise, too. It makes sense to try and find an exercise you enjoy, as this means that you will be more likely to keep doing the activity. It can also be helpful to do an activity that brings you into contact with other people, such as a team sport like football or tennis. By including regular exercise as part of your daily routine, you may make new friends as well as improving your physical fitness, sleep cycle and energy levels.

If you have not exercised in quite a few years, check with your doctor before embarking on a new exercise programme.

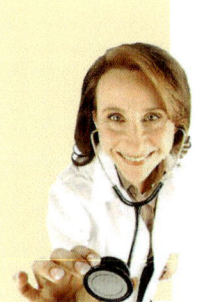

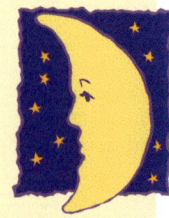

Good Sleep Habits

Having a regular sleep routine make it more likely that you will have a good night's sleep, wake up feeling refreshed, and be less tired during the day.

Good sleep habits include:
- ☐ Making sure you have a calm bedroom which is dark and quiet.

- ☐ Get into the habit of going to bed at the same time each day and getting up at the same time.

- ☐ Just use your bedroom to sleep in and do not watch television in bed. This will mean that you begin to associate lying in bed with going to sleep.

- ☐ Try to get into the habit of doing something you find relaxing before you go to bed. Suggestions include taking a warm bath, listening to calming music or doing relaxation exercises.

- ☐ Don't eat large meals late at night.

- ☐ Avoid drinking tea or coffee, eating chocolate or smoking before going to bed

- ☐ Don't drink alcohol before going to bed.

- ☐ Avoid sleeping in the day after 4pm.

- ☐ Try not to start thinking about difficulties and problem just prior to going to bed. If you do start to worry about particular things write them down and tell yourself that you will deal with them in the morning when you have more energy.

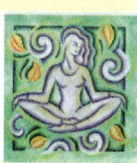

[26]

7

Finally…

Hopefully, this leaflet has given you some ideas to help manage your fatigue. Some of the ideas may be more helpful than others but give yourself time to try them out to see what best works for you.

GETTING A GOOD NIGHT'S SLEEP

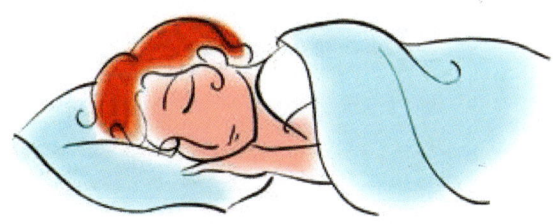

How do I get off to sleep?

1. **General Habits.** Get regular exercise. Eat a balanced diet, and try to avoid being overweight. Do not smoke - cut down if you do smoke. Avoid excessive alcohol. Stay clear of illicit drugs. Note the side-effects of any medications that you are taking, in case they affect your sleep.

   Try not to drink too much coffee during the day. Set aside part of the day to deal with issues that cause you stress. Depression and anxiety may have major effects on sleep, so make sure that you get help and advice regarding these. Discuss with your doctor any medical factors, such as hormone changes, urinary problems or painful conditions, that may keep you awake.

   If possible, apart from a quick nap do not sleep for any period during the day. Have a regular time for going to bed, and a regular time for waking up. Your sleep may be affected if you are working and have to work long hours or night-shifts, if you have a stressful job, or if you do a lot of travelling as part of your daily routine.

   If you play computer games late at night or listen to fast-beat music, this may also affect your sleep. Keeping a diary of your good and bad sleep days may help to find a pattern that gives you clues to work on.

2. **Your bed and bedroom.** Make sure your bed and pillow are comfortable. Ensure that there is not too much light or noise coming into the room.

   Avoid having a television, radio or computer in the room. If do you have a computer or television in your room, avoid leaving them on throughout the night. Make sure your bed and your bedroom are not too hot or too cold, and that your night clothes are comfortable.

3. **Before you go to bed.** Avoid any heavy meal or much alcohol in the hours before you go to bed, but a light snack is fine. Do not drink lots of fluid in the 1-2 hours before you go to bed, as you are more likely to want to wake up in the middle of the night to go to the toilet.

   Do not smoke or drink coffee shortly before going to bed, but a warm milky drink with a light snack may be a useful habit to try. It can help to unwind and relax in the hour before you go to bed – perhaps listen to gentle music. You could also watch goldfish for 10-15 minutes, either real fish in a bowl or an artificial display on a computer screen.

   Some people find that it helps to regularly have a hot shower before they go to bed. Try to get into a standard routine in the hour before you go to bed, as your mind will associate this routine with a good night's sleep. If you are not at all tired near bed-time, wait for a little while till you do feel tired.

4. When in bed. Avoid watching TV, eating, listening to the radio, using your mobile phone, or working on a laptop computer when you are in bed. Keep your bed for sleeping – this may also help you fall asleep. If you have a partner, and he / she is affecting your sleep, for example by snoring, see if their problem can be treated, otherwise you may find you have to sleep in separate rooms.

How do I get back to sleep if I wake up in the middle of the night or early in the morning?

1. Find a reason. If there is a specific reason for waking up, try to deal with the cause of this….if you have to go the toilet, are in pain, are too cold or too hot, have things on your mind, etc see if you can find ways for dealing with this. If you have particular worries on your mind, write them down on a pen and pad that you could keep next to your bedside, and deal with them the next day.

2. Relax. Do not panic if you wake up in the middle of the night. Stay calm, and try to relax for 20-30 minutes. This may take the form of saying reassuring things to yourself – that you *will* get back to sleep in a short while, taking deep breaths, picturing a relaxing scene, humming a relaxing tune to yourself, etc.

If you wake up less than a couple of hours before your normal waking time, it may be best to carry on with you normal morning routine and spend part of the morning doing some light reading, listening to music or watching TV. If you find that exercise relaxes you, then you might think of going for an early morning jog.

3. Try things that have worked in the past. If after 20-30 minutes you are still awake, you could get up for a short while, and do anything that in the past has helped you get off to sleep at night – having a warm drink and light snack, listening to soft music, having a hot shower, etc.

This leaflet was produced on the basis of clinical experience and published research. The advice in this leaflet needs to be considered in the context of each person's individual circumstances, and other treatment they may be receiving.

ADVICE FOR PEOPLE WHO ARE RETURNING TO WORK AFTER HAVING SUFFERED A BRAIN INJURY OR BRAIN ILLNESS

When you have recovered enough from your brain injury or brain illness to think about going back to work, it is important to bear a few things in mind.

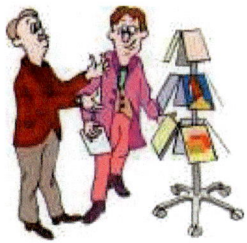

1. *GUIDANCE* - Seek expert guidance from health professionals and support services at work. The ideas presented in this leaflet are intended to supplement the advice you receive from these sources.

2. *FATIGUE* - It may be some time since you last worked and you will almost certainly find that although whilst you were still at home you felt fit and well and able to cope, when you actually go back to work you will get tired more easily. This can be especially so in the first few days and weeks of returning to work. Be ready to take a break if you feel you are getting tired or if you are finding it hard to concentrate.

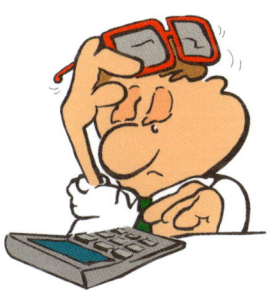

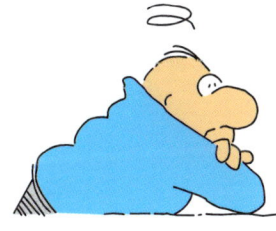

3. *PRESSURE* - You may also find that, because of tiredness and frustrations, you are feeling more anxious than you did before your brain injury or brain illness. Try to cope with any frustrations or anxiety by staying calm, and by seeking advice where necessary.

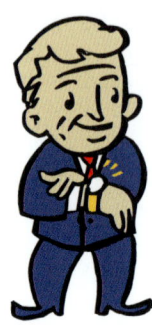 4. *STAMINA* - Make sure you monitor the amount of time you spend at work. You may have been working an eight- or nine-hour day before your brain illness or brain injury, but you almost certainly will not be able to work that long a day when you initially return to work. You will need to slowly build up to this.

5. *TIME* - Try to make sure you don't have lots of time pressures on your work. To begin with, you may need to allow yourself more time to carry out tasks, even if you were able to do them quickly before.

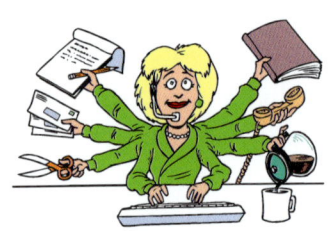 6. *OVERLOAD* - It may be helpful to make sure you only do one job at a time to begin with. Doing lots of tasks at the same time can be very demanding and you may find you gradually need to build up to this.

7. *COMPLEXITY* - To begin with, try to keep the tasks that you do at work fairly straightforward and simple. As you settle into the routine of working again, and begin to get your confidence back, gradually increase the complexity of the tasks that you do.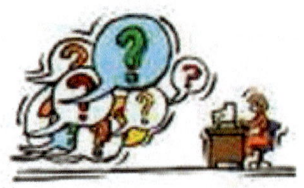

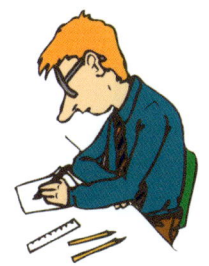
8. *FAMILIARITY* - New tasks may be more difficult to perform than ones you were very familiar with before. Try to begin by doing tasks that you are very familiar with. When learning new tasks make sure you give yourself time to practise or make notes of what you have to do.

9. *SUPPORT* - Support from work colleagues can be important so that you can get help when you need it. Try to ensure that you have such support in place so that it is there if you need it. To those people who matter, briefly explain what has happened to you and the way you are going to phase your return to work.
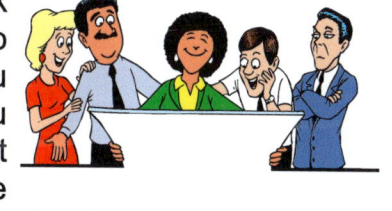

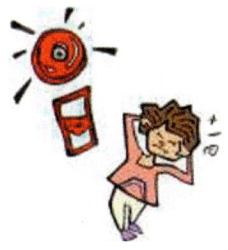
10. *DISTRACTIONS* - When you go back to work, if at all possible try to work in a quiet environment – some people find that noise from others talking or from machines can disrupt their concentration.

11. *PROGRESS* - If you gradually increase your workload, keeping in mind the factors mentioned above, you should find that your confidence also steadily improves. If you find that you do get into difficulties, or if you have any problems coping, remember that you can always contact health professionals to get further advice and support.
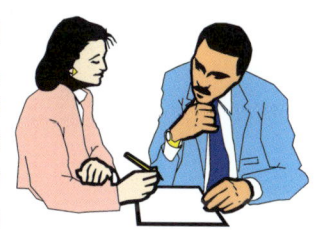

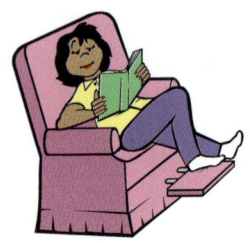

12. *REST* - When you are not at work try to get plenty of rest and relaxation, and try to make sure that you get a good night's sleep. Find time to take part in hobbies and pastimes that you find easy and enjoyable.

Study Tips

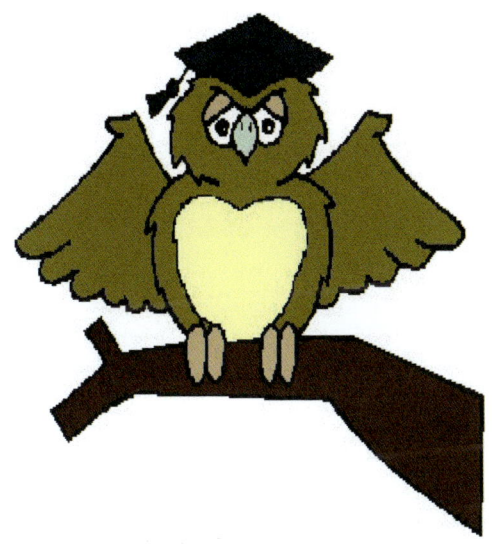

Study Skills for Students

Read this booklet a few times a year, and especially when you are preparing for exams, so that you remember to do the right things.

Be well organised! There are three areas in which you can be well organised – your time, your room and your personal belongings.

Organise Your Time

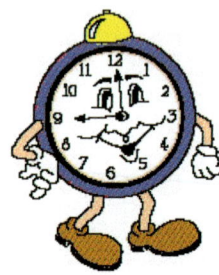
It is useful to have a well planned routine. Arrange your week so that you allow for set times and days for homework and for revision. Plan your revision well in advance. A regular amount of revision each week is better than cramming it all in at the last minute.

A weekly timetable is a useful way of doing this. You could attach this to a magnetic whiteboard or to a wall.

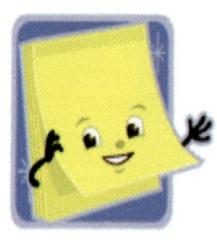
You can also plan your time for a study session using Post-It Notes. You could use them to write down set times for starting and finishing particular topics. The more precise you are when you are planning your work, the easier it will be to get things done.

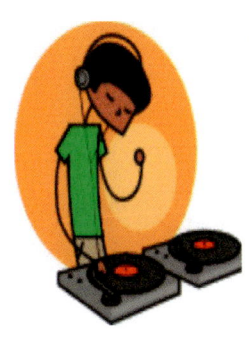

Be realistic in your revision plans, do not over-commit yourself. When planning your time, fit in regular breaks for relaxing and hobbies. Try not to revise when you are tired or upset.

Minimise distractions when you are revising – tell others so that you will not be interrupted, turn off your mobile phone, TV, radio, etc.

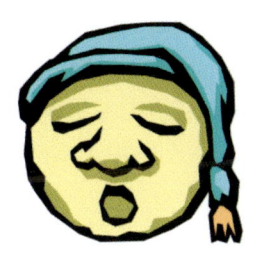

In general, earlier in the day is better for revising than late in the evening. Although you may find yourself occasionally working late into the night, make that the exception rather than the rule.

Try to revise in the same place at the same time so that revising becomes a natural habit.

Organise Your Study Area

A tidy well-organised room can help to improve your studying.

Try to keep your study area clutter-free.

Keep things in set places, and get into the habit of putting things away after you have used them. Label drawers and folders. This will save you wasting time trying to find things.

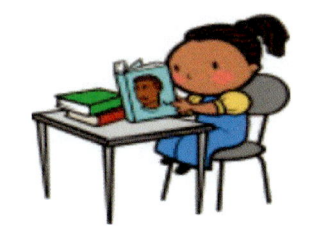

[38]

Having a magnetic whiteboard or noticeboard near your study area may help too. You can use this to write down important things that you have to remember, e.g. chemical formulae or foreign language words.

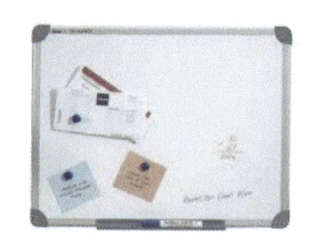

Organise Your Personal Belongings

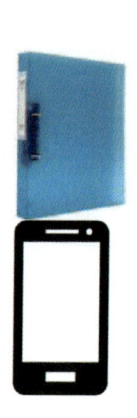

If you have a college bag, make sure it is organised and not in a mess. Have name tags on your belongings so that they can be returned to you if you lose them.

You may find it helpful to have a ring folder for keeping class notes or class / lecture handouts.

If you keep notes on your mobile phone, try and have those notes synchronised with your computer / tablet so that you can easily view them and make any changes.

Make Good Notes

Before attending a lecture, it is useful to read some background information about the topic. Having a summary in your mind helps your brain to better absorb what you will be hearing when you attend the lecture.

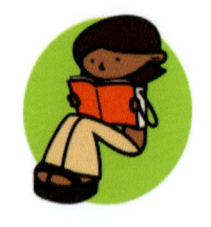

If you make notes during a lecture, try to write them in your own words.

If there is no handout of the content of the lecture, and you have problems in keeping up with what is said, see if you can record the lecture on a mobile phone or voice recorder, after getting permission from the teacher / lecturer.

Some bits of software, such as Dragon, can enable recorded speech to be automatically transcribed into text. Electronic pens such as LiveScribe perform a similar function.

Try Mind Maps

Try and organize a topic you are revising into ways that break it up into meaningful parts.

Try and find or draw a 'mind-map' or diagram that summarises the topic you are revising – this could be like a tree with branches, or a wheel with spokes, or large 'moons' connected to smaller moons.

Try and make links between different parts that you have created in your 'mind-map', so that when you think of one part the other part will also come to mind.

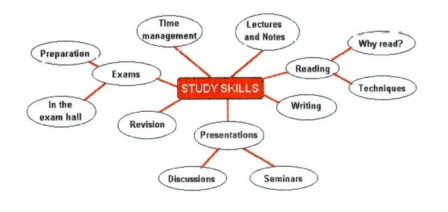

[40]

Use Memory Tricks

Memory tricks ('mnemonics') involve making links or associations that make the information easier to recall on a later occasion.

For example, if you had to remember that the ozone layer in the atmosphere consists of **Manmade** and **Natural** pollution, you could take the first letters of these two words, **M** and **N**, and then think of the sweets called **M & Ns** as a 'memory trick' to help you remember this. You could also picture **M** and **N** sweets falling from the sky to remind you of the ozone layer in the atmosphere!

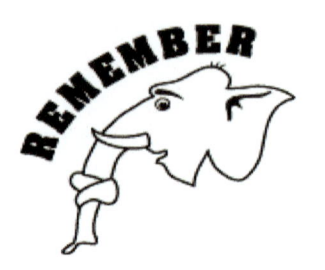

Do Mini Mocks

Test yourself regularly ('mini mocks') for things you have revised. Bringing items to mind again and again over increasing intervals will help you remember them better.

A good trick is to write as much as you can about a topic on a ruled sheet of paper. If you used a mind-map or something similar when revising, try and use this to help you remember what to write. When you have finished, fill in the bits you missed with a red pen. You should remember more each time you try!

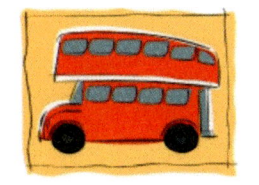

'Recall and Review' is where you test yourself and then re-read the original to see what you have forgotten. You could set yourself reminders on your mobile phone to prompt you to use this technique.

If you regularly try and recall things you have revised, even when you are sitting in a bus or having a shower, this will help the items stick in your memory.

Have Good Exam Techniques

Make sure you get a good night's sleep before the exam.

Read the questions carefully. Underline key words. Plan your answers. Work out how much time you will spend answering each question.

It may help to picture the room where you revised the topic in question, or the books/notes that you read at the time.

If one question is very difficult, start with other questions you can do more easily and allow enough time to come back to the difficult one at the end.

If you can't find a word or name you are thinking of, going through the letters of the alphabet may help.

Try and think of any mind-maps you made or memory tricks you used.

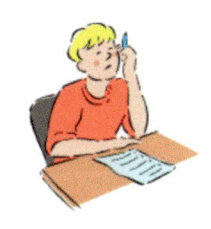

TOP STUDY TIPS
(Keep this Summary on your wall / whiteboard for the duration of your studies and look at it now and again)

- ✓ Revise little and often. Plan your revision months in advance rather than leaving things to the last minute.
- ✓ Organize your time each day and each week so that you set aside time for homework and revision in a distraction-free environment.
- ✓ Use reminders on your smartphone to help you be well organized with your time.
- ✓ Make sure your workspace is well-organized. Think of using magnetic whiteboards or wall-calendars.
- ✓ Use mind-maps and other ways of organizing what you have to learn to help it make more sense and stick better in your mind.
- ✓ Use any 'memory tricks' or association techniques to help you remember key words or headings.
- ✓ Regularly test yourself for what you have recently learned ('mini mocks'). Set reminders to help you do this. If possible, also have 'Recall and Review' sessions where you test yourself and also then review what it is you did not recall, so that you can concentrate more on these bits, making links between them and the bits you did recall.
- ✓ Look after your well-being. Deal with any fatigue and sleep issues, and take time to relax.

Looking After Someone Who Is Confused
A Carer's Guide

This booklet has been written to help those looking after people who have major memory and concentration problems, usually as the result of a brain illness or brain injury. We have used the word 'confused' to describe these individuals, although this term often means different things to different people. By 'confused', we would include difficulties such as – cannot remember what is happening from one day to the next, and often from one minute to the next; repeatedly asking the day of the week; getting lost easily and frequently in very familiar places; and not being able to do even simple tasks around the home that were once easy to do. This booklet suggests ways in which a carer could help someone with confusion remain safe and cope better in everyday situations.

Safety First

- Make a note of potentially risky areas for the person, such as in the bathroom or the kitchen. If there are any hazards, try to reduce the likelihood of harm, or remove the hazard where possible.

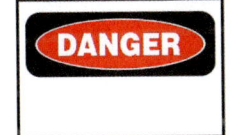

- Put away things that could be dangerous or cause harm, such as sharp instruments, power tools etc.

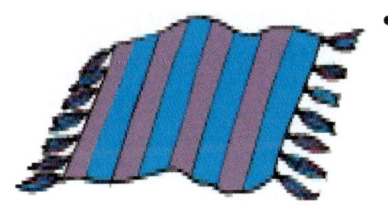

- To reduce the risk of falls, make sure that floor coverings are secure and that mats are not frayed. Make sure that things are not left lying around on the floor and keep floors dry. If necessary, reduce the amount of furniture that is around.

- Turn the thermostat on the water heater down to reduce the risk of the person scalding him or herself.

- If there is an open fire, or heater with exposed elements, always use a fireguard.

- If there is a danger that the person may take too many tablets at once, use a pillbox with different compartments and only put out enough medicine for one day at a time.

Be organised

- Make sure that the place where the person lives is tidy and well organised, with items in fixed places. Keep things such as clothes, items in the kitchen, items in the bathroom, etc in the same, regular place.

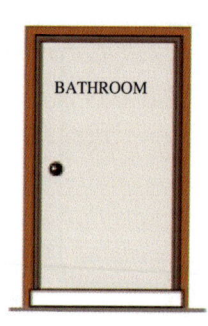

- Put labels or pictures on cupboards or drawers to give the person an idea of what is inside. You can also put labels or pictures on doors of particular rooms, for example, the bathroom. Make the labels or pictures large enough so that they are easily seen. If some doors have distinctive colours, this may also help the person to remember what the room is used for.

- For some activities such as dressing, making a simple meal or drink, using the phone, etc you may find that you have to make up an 'instruction sheet', with the steps of what to do clearly written out and displayed in a handy place.

[45]

Have a regular routine

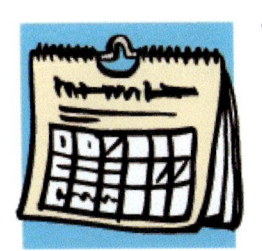

- Try to keep to a regular routine each day, with things happening at the same times each day or each week. This will help to avoid situations where the person may forget to do something. The timing of events and activities is not as important as the order in which they occur. For example, if the person always gets out of bed, has breakfast, then bathes and dresses, it is not a good idea to change the routine and have them get out of bed, bathe and dress and then have breakfast.

- Get to know when the person's 'best time of day' is. This will often be in the morning, when they are feeling fresh, but if they do not sleep well it may be later in the day. Where possible, try to arrange appointments, visits and other activities during their best time of day.

- Plan activities that are of short duration and include breaks. Try not to do too much in one day, since you may find that the person tires easily.

- For some activities such as dressing or making a simple meal/drink, you may find it useful to make up an 'instruction sheet', with the steps clearly written out and displayed in a handy place.

Keep the person oriented

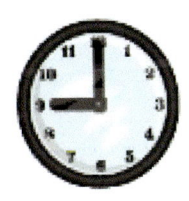

- If the person is always asking the time of day or day of the week, consider placing a day-date clock in a prominent place and remind them to look at it. Clocks displaying only the day of the week are also available.

- Alternatively, if he/she wears a watch with the day and date displayed on it, prompt the person to look at their watch.

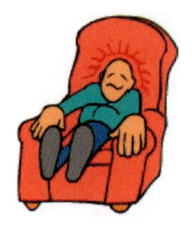

- When the person has a rest during the day, sit them in an easy chair or sofa rather than in bed, so that when they wake up they know it was from a nap rather than a night's sleep. If the person is resting near a window, the daylight will also help orient them to the time of the day.

- If the person keeps asking for information such as where they are, this could be written on a white-board in large, clear lettering and put in a convenient, easy-to-see place. If the person has a weekly schedule for things that are done on certain days, have this schedule clearly displayed. You can also use a white-board to write down important events for each day, or about particular things that are going to happen in the future, e.g. people who are due to visit.

- If there is a safety checklist for things to be done last thing at night, have this displayed in a prominent place in the person's bedroom.

- In some situations, it may be useful to have information readily visible to the person on a wristband. For example, if the person repeatedly asks for information such as what is wrong with them or where they are, they could be told to look at their wristband. Their address and home telephone number could also be written there in case they get lost.

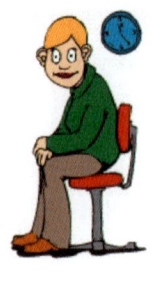

- Try not to tell the person about things that are going to happen too far in advance. People who are confused may have problems planning ahead. They may become upset or worried if they think they have missed something or will forget something.

[47]

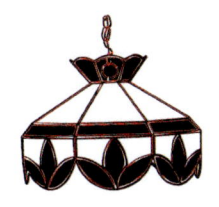

- Leave a light on in the hallway at night. Waking during the night and not being able to see anything familiar can be quite frightening, particularly for someone who is confused.

- If you are going out, write a note saying where you are going, with a contact name, address and telephone number. Put the note in a prominent place where it will be clearly seen.

- Most people who are confused may be unable to use a standard mobile phone, but simpler phones are now available. If the person is using a mobile phone, you could try and programme reminders that go off at key times, or send them text messages as reminders. In the case of land-line phones, 'photophones' which have pre-dial buttons with photographs of the person being called are also now available.

- It may be useful to keep a 'memory book' to record important events that have happened each day. You could consider inserting some photographs of outings. The front or back of the book could also contain information that is needed in an emergency. Encourage the person to look at this memory book each day as part of their routine. If you think the person is interested in the news and can take in the information, then you could give them a daily newspaper of their choice, or have a TV news channel regularly on.

Feeling useful and valued is important

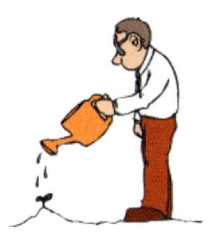

- Enabling the person to help out with simple tasks around the house such as dusting, setting the table, sorting the laundry, or watering the garden, may give them a sense of purpose.

- Exercise is also important, so if possible try to take the person out for a walk or some other form of exercise (e.g. swimming) at least two or three times a week.

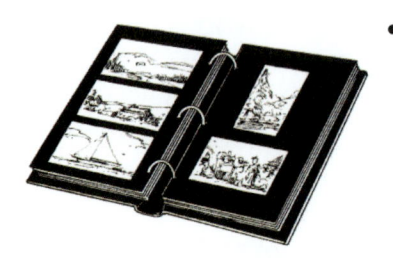

- Encourage skills and activities that are easy and pleasurable for the person to take part in. Consider past hobbies or interests that they were good at, listening to music they like, watching videos that engage their interest, looking at familiar photographs, or being in the company of children or pets in a safe setting. Having a favourite piece of music in the background may help to make the person feel better. In some instances, this may help calm them and make them more co-operative.

- Do things to remind the person that they are valued and loved, even if this just means touching and embracing them from time to time.

- Have a pencil and notepad or Post-It Note Dispenser near to the telephone so that the person can write down any messages that he or she receives. It may be useful to also have a prompt card stuck somewhere, with key advice such as – **'Write all messages down. Tell the caller that you are writing the message down. Ask the caller for their name and telephone number. Read back the message to the caller'**.

Handle conversations carefully

- People who are confused may have problems in understanding what has been said to them or in remembering what they have been told. You may find yourself needing to repeat something several times or having to write things down. Although often frustrating, try to be patient and understanding when repeating information.

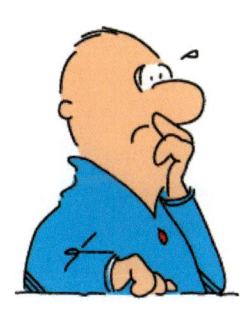

- The conversations that you have with the person may, on occasions, be 'muddled'. If what they say does not make sense, gently try to change the topic to something the person finds interesting and meaningful. If the patient insists on you saying something in response, it is best to try to give a neutral reply.

- If, during a conversation, the person becomes angry or upset, try to distract them rather than argue with them.

- In general, try to follow three rules – avoid asking questions, generally agree with what the person is saying, and try not to interrupt the person during a conversation or while they are doing something.

- If the person is erroneously re-living a period in the past, or making up events that have happened or might happen ('confabulation') it is usually fine to go along with that rather than confront the person with the reality of the present. You need not feel guilty about doing this. Try to address any concerns that underlie the confabulation. Try to cover the topic indirectly from another angle. It may help to distract the person to other topics or activities they find interesting and enjoyable.

- When you say something, keep the information short with one item at a time. If it is a request or a message, ask the person to repeat it back in their own words to make sure that they have heard and understood it properly.

Make good use of past memories

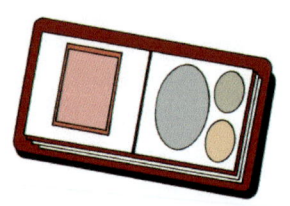

- 'Confused' people may have difficulty remembering some of their past and may also be uncertain about the identity of close family members. One-to-one interaction with familiar family members will help. If that is not possible, keeping familiar items, such as family photographs or family members' personal belongings around them may help. In some instances, it may be helpful to play a video of a past family occasion where the person was present, and which they remember and relate to.

- If the person is regularly asking about relatives or friends, especially if they are unsure whether the person is still alive, it may help to have photographs on view (e.g. on a wall or mantel-piece), with names and ages written if necessary.

- Try not to keep 'quizzing' the person in an attempt to test their memory. For example, asking 'Do you remember her?' 'What is her name?' and so on. This can make the person feel anxious or that they have failed. It is best just to indicate the person's name to gently remind them.

Stay calm and in control when dealing with outbursts of anger

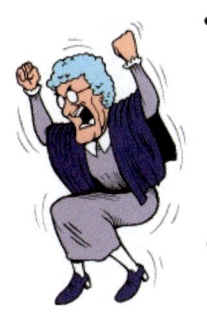

- The person may feel angry about the situation they find themselves in. Do not take this anger personally – it is always easier for the person to 'lash out' at someone close, even though that person is not the cause of their anger.

- Try to find out if there is any pattern as to when and why anger outbursts occur. By identifying and avoiding situations that lead to these outbursts, you may be able to prevent their occurrence.

- If possible, distract the person's attention towards another activity that they find interesting or calming, or remove the person from the upsetting situation.

- Be calm and firm - encourage and support the person to use more positive ways to deal and cope with similar situations.

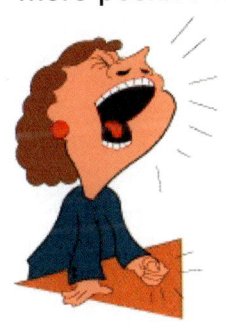

- If there is an outburst of anger and you are unable to determine the cause or to distract the person, try not to retaliate. Instead make sure that the person is safe from harm and leave them alone to calm down. When you return, the outburst will probably be over, and they may have forgotten the trigger for their anger.

[52]

Prevent the person from wandering

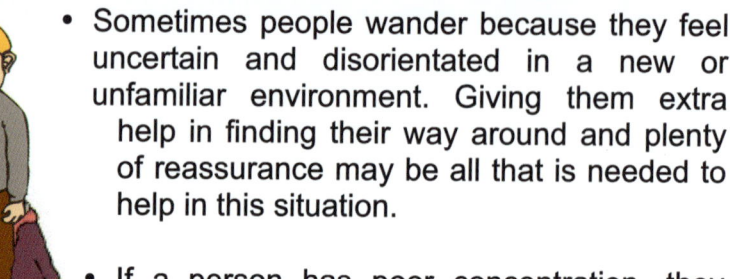

- Sometimes people wander because they feel uncertain and disorientated in a new or unfamiliar environment. Giving them extra help in finding their way around and plenty of reassurance may be all that is needed to help in this situation.

- If a person has poor concentration, they may become easily distracted and also more likely to wander.

- Some wandering may also occur due to loss of short-term memory. For example, the person may go off to the bathroom, and simply forget where it was they were going.

- People sometimes wander off searching for someone or something related to their past. The best way to deal with this type of wandering is not to reason with the person but instead gently distract their attention and bring them back home.

- Another, often overlooked, reason for wandering is that the person is in some sort of physical discomfort or pain that is eased by walking. It is important therefore, to try and find out if they are experiencing any physical problem or pain and to remedy it if possible.

- It is usually wise not to confront a person who is determined to leave the house, as they may then become very upset. Instead, try accompanying them a little way and then diverting their attention so that you can return home together.

- If a person does wander off alone, try not to show anger or anxiety when you do find them. Reassure them and try to get

[53]

them back into familiar surroundings and into a familiar routine as quickly as possible.

- Ensure that the person has details of their home address and a contact phone number with them at all times. Where possible, providing them with an easy-to-use mobile phone for use in situations when they are away from home, will help with keeping in touch.

- Make sure that friends and neighbours are aware of the possibility that the person may wander off so that they can help to keep an eye out for them.

- Electronic alarm systems that will trigger when someone approaches a door or when a door is opened are available on the market. These can give you an early warning that the person is about to leave the house. There are also companies that offer tracking systems which can help you to locate someone.

Don't be too hard on yourself

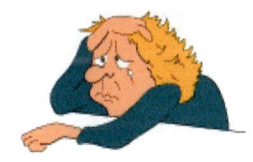

- Feeling angry or upset are natural responses to stressful situations. Don't be too hard on yourself if you feel angry as a result of the stresses and strains of taking on the role of carer.

- Expect a certain amount of family conflict during the time that you have a confused person to look after. Each family member will experience different emotions and will have different demands placed on them when someone else in the family is confused. Try to make time for each other and to talk through any problems together.

- Gently introduce any unfamiliar helpers to the person suffering from confusion and try to establish a routine with that new helper.

- If there is anything that you do not understand about the person's memory loss, their illness or the treatment that they are being given, don't be afraid to ask a doctor or other professional.

- Remember that you are not alone. There are a number of support groups and other organizations that can give you help and advice and provide a 'listening ear'. Nursing staff and other care workers will be able to give you details of these groups and organizations.

- Finally, remember that being the relative, carer or friend of a confused person can be stressful. If you can get help with domestic or other activities, then do accept that help! Most importantly, be sure to take care of your own health. Schedule 'time out' to have a break and remember to look after yourself!

RESOURCES ON THE INTERNET

There are a number of websites that provide helpful information on looking after someone who is confused, where to buy memory aids, etc. A listing of these can be found on –

www.londonmemoryclinic.com

Please keep in mind that this booklet is not meant to be a substitute for professional advice or treatment.

Word Finding Tips

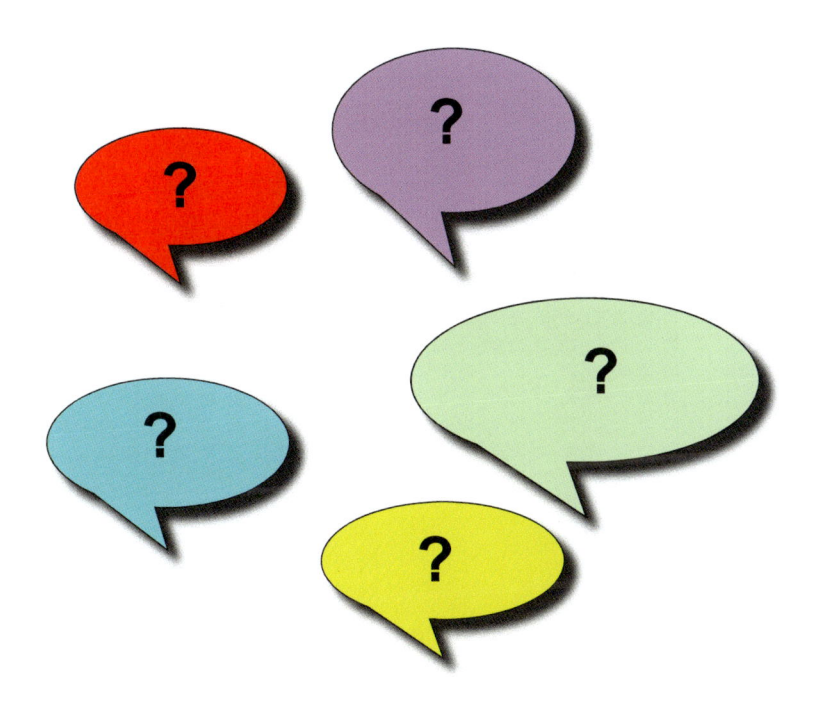

Stay calm

It will be more difficult to find a word if you panic. Stay calm and say reassuring things such as…'It'll come back to me in a moment'.

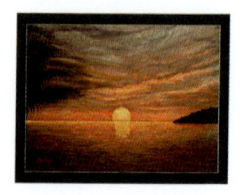

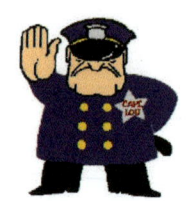

Think of associations and pause

Think of associations to the word you cannot find, or to the person/object whose name you cannot remember, and wait for a while - the word may come to you after a few minutes.

Think of a similar word

If you cannot think of the word you are looking for, you may find it easier to think of another word that could take its place in the sentence – e.g. substitute 'anonymous' with 'unknown'.

Replace the word with a short phrase

Sometimes it is difficult to find a substitute word. In these instances it may be easier to express yourself using a short phrase instead – e.g. replace 'inexcusable' with 'it was not the right thing to do'.

Go through the letters of the alphabet

You can try and find the word you are looking for by going through each letter of the alphabet. This may be particularly helpful when you are trying to recall someone's name.

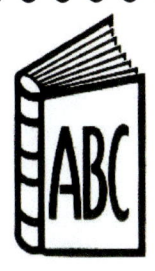

Ask someone else

If there is someone handy you can ask, remember you could always look to that person to help you out.

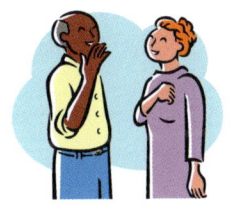

Stay confident

It may be useful to have in reserve a few phrases that you always rely on in social situations where you get stuck for a word – e.g. confidently saying 'Do you know the word has escaped me!'. You can also make light of the lapse – e.g. 'My little grey cells must have gone on strike!'

Play word games

You may find it helpful to play word games like Scrabble or simple cross-word puzzles. This will give you the opportunity to practice your word-finding skills and the techniques that you can use when you get stuck for a word. Having to look up a dictionary or thesaurus may indirectly help to increase your vocabulary, making it easier for you to think of other words when you are stuck for a particular word.

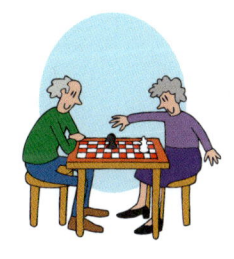

Over ➢

[58]

Ways to avoid having word-finding difficulties in the first place

- Try to avoid getting into lengthy conversations when you are feeling tired or anxious, or if you have had a few drinks of alcohol.

- Avoid talking a lot when you have other things on your mind, or when you are trying to do something else at the same time.

- Try to use simple, short sentences in a conversation.

- If you can, rehearse what it is you are going to say.

- Have breaks between sentences to help gather your thoughts.

- Slow down your rate of speech…..the faster you talk, the more likely you are to come across word-finding difficulties.

- Try to stick to talking about familiar things…..if you find yourself having to talk for the first time about something that is unfamiliar to you, or which you have not talked about before, practise several times what you are going to say, and have notes at hand.

ADVICE FOR WARD STAFF DEALING WITH CONFUSED AND AGITATED PATIENTS

Professor Narinder Kapur

BRAIN DAMAGE AND BEHAVIOUR

Points to remember -

- Sensory or physical handicaps, impairments or damage may affect cognitive and behavioural functioning - e.g. hearing, visual loss, loss of sense of smell. Cognitive functioning may also be affected by other, non-specific, factors - e.g. increased tiredness.

- In addition to physical limitations, a damaged brain can result in disturbances of cognitive function, mood, temperament and behaviour

- Be aware of the main cognitive, mood and behavioural deficits after damage to particular brain regions, and consider these as they apply to each particular patient.

- A damaged brain, together with the fact that the patient is in an unfamiliar environment, may result in further abnormalities of behaviour - e.g. poor memory, perseveration, confabulation, hallucinations, fear, anger, impaired comprehension, etc.

- The brain-injured patient may have more cognitive deficits than he or she is aware of.

- Many severe behavioural and cognitive problems in the early stages of recovery are temporary and will spontaneously resolve over a few days. In addition, they may be secondary to factors such as clinical/sub-clinical epileptic activity, drug toxicity, etc.

ASSESSMENT

- Patients who are severely cognitively impaired, or those with severe physical or communication handicaps can be assessed by using forced-choice recognition tests for reading and identifying pictures (i.e. patients are shown words and/or pictures and then later asked to pick the ones that they have seen before from a set containing those words and/or pictures that they have seen and some that they have not), and by the use of gestures to explain instructions. Scales such as the Wessex Head Injury Matrix may be useful for those who have recovered from a comatose state but are not yet mobile or unable to communicate verbally.

- Inconsistencies in test performance, behaviour that is not usually associated with neurological conditions and the possibility of some secondary gain by the patient, can be indicative of psychogenic conditions such as hysteria or malingering. In suspected cases, provide a way out for patient to 'recover' so that he or she does not lose face.

- Remember, the patient is in a new and unfamiliar environment, surrounded by strangers. Furthermore, he or she may not know why they are there.

- Keep a well-organised environment with particular things in particular places.

- Provide marked routes to the toilet and bathroom, and labels or pictures on doors to specific rooms can help prevent the patient getting lost.

- Keep familiar stimuli, such as photographs of family or friends, near the bedside.

- Have a well-structured routine, with set things happening at set times.

- Avoid making unnecessary changes to the environment or routine.

- Keep noise to a minimum, particularly for patients who have suffered a head injury.

INTERACTIONS

- Give the patient plenty of reassurance.
- Ensure that the patient is allowed plenty of rest time.
- Keep a *Personal Profile Sheet* with the patient's details (names of family and friends, pets, interests, etc) at the end of the bed.
- As far as possible, try to maintain continuity of staff members who deal with the patient.

- Try to give your name to the patient when initiating conversation. Make sure your name-badge is clearly visible.
- Limit the number of visitors he or she has at one time.
- Avoid overloading the patient with information or asking questions that are too cognitively demanding.
- In general, try to follow three rules – avoid asking questions, generally agree with what the person is saying, and try not to interrupt the person during a conversation or while they are doing something.
- If the person is erroneously re-living a period in the past, or making up events that have happened or might happen ('confabulation') it is usually fine to go along with that rather than confront the person with the reality of the present. You need not feel guilty about doing this. Try to address any concerns that underlie the confabulation. Try to cover the topic indirectly from another angle. It may help to distract the person to other topics or activities they find interesting and enjoyable.
- Keep the patient's family informed about their condition, their treatment and any therapy programmes.

ACTIVITIES

- Concentrate on skills that the patient can do and things that he or she enjoys.
- Try to avoid situations where the patient makes lots of mistakes. Set realistic goals. Have initial goals fairly modest so that the patient may experience success and reinforcement from the beginning
- Break up large tasks into smaller parts and provide verbal or physical support. These cues and prompts can then be gradually reduced.
- Give the patient encouragement and/or reward as appropriate for successfully completed tasks.

HELPING MEMORY & ORIENTATION

- Especially in the early stages after severe brain injury, patients may have difficulty in retaining what has been told to them, and may also have problems in understanding speech. Repeating information several times, and using multiple modalities (speech, writing, pictures,) may help in this respect.

- Have the time, day, month, year, and place clearly displayed so that this information can be seen by the patient. Clocks and watches are available that have time and date information. It may help to have a magnetic white board on a nearby wall, with key reminders written on the board with a marker pen, or on Post-It tape in large print. If you think the person is interested in the news and can take in the information, then you could give them a daily newspaper of their choice, or have a TV news channel regularly on.

- You could make up a wristband for the patient. This should have their name on, very brief details of what has happened to them and/or what is wrong with them, how long they have been in hospital and answers to any other frequently asked questions. When the patient asks what is wrong with them or where they are, encourage them to look at their wristband.

- Have a paper and pencil handy at the patient's bedside so that the patient can write things down rather than rely on their memory.

- Keep a communication notebook so that staff and visitors can record the day and time of their interactions with the patient.

- 'Confused' patients may also have lost many of their past memories and may even be unable to recognize close family members. While such amnesia is usually temporary, having reminders available (e.g. family photographs) may help such memories to return. Some patients may respond to favourite music from the past – this may not only bring back past memories, but also be a useful distraction when the person is upset or agitated for some reason.

MANAGEMENT OF PROBLEM BEHAVIOUR

- An accurate assessment of the problem behaviour or problem mood-state will help successful management. Understanding why a behaviour is occurring (cause) needs to precede attempts at treatment (cure).

- Cognitive and behavioural deficits may influence each other. Cognitive deficits may lead to frustration and depression. Comprehension problems may result in the patient getting confused about interventions or treatments. Memory problems may lead to conflict about what was said or not said. Expressive difficulties may result in frustration and the patient being misunderstood by staff. Behavioural problems, anxiety or depression may result in poor concentration and then other impairments such as memory deficits

- A logical approach to problem behaviours can help, though this may require the involvement of a psychologist. Try to determine the 'A-B-C' of the problem behaviour. What preceded the behaviour (**A** - 'Antecedents') for example, the state of patient, events in the environment, etc., what are the features of the behaviour itself and how often does it occur (**B** - 'Behaviour') and (iii) what follows the behaviour (**C** - 'Consequences'). This will help to determine the nature of the problem behaviour.

- If possible, quantify behaviour in order to have an objective baseline with which to monitor improvement/deterioration. Essentially, determine how often the behavioural disturbance occurs (you may wish to break down the behaviour into different parts).

- Find out what incentives or rewards the patient has responded to in the past. These may be verbal (praise), leisure-related (watching TV, having a cigarette), food or drink related, or money-related. Reward good behaviour, provide appropriate feedback to inappropriate behaviour. This may involve provision or removal of privileges or tangible rewards. Remember to show the patient examples of appropriate behaviour if this does not spontaneously occur.

- *Anger Outbursts* – Carry out an accurate assessment of when and why anger outbursts occur. Try to identify and to avoid situations that lead to these in first place, thus preventing their occurrence. Try not to make any direct 'knee-jerk' response - distract the patient's attention to another activity, remove the patient from the situation or remove yourself from the situation. Be calm and firm, giving appropriate feedback as to adverse consequences of behaviour and encourage and support more positive ways that the patient can use to deal with similar situations. Do not take anger personally.

- *Socially Inappropriate Behaviour/Speech* – Use a procedure similar to that detailed above in response to anger outbursts. On the first few occasions give feedback and suggest alternative ways of behaving. Subsequently ignore inappropriate behaviour.

- Try to maintain consistency in the management of a patient's problem behaviour between staff (day/night, nurses and others), and between family members.

WANDERING

- Ensure that the patient has at least two nametags attached to them that give details of the ward they are on and a contact phone number.

- Make sure that other ward staff are aware of the possibility that patients may wander off so that they can keep an eye out for them.

- Sometimes patients wander because they feel uncertain and disorientated in a new and unfamiliar environment. Giving them extra help in finding their way around and plenty of reassurance may be all that is needed in this type of situation.

- Some wandering may occur due to the loss of short-term memory that occurs following brain injury. The patient may go off somewhere, for example, to the bathroom, and simply forget where it was they were going.

- Patients sometimes wander off searching for someone or something related to their past. The best way to deal with this type of wandering is not to reason, but to gently distract their attention and bring them back to the ward.

- Another, often overlooked, reason for wandering is that the patient is in some sort of physical discomfort or pain which is eased by walking. It is important therefore, to try and find out if there is any physical problem/source of pain and to alleviate it if possible.

- It is usually wise not to confront a patient who is determined to leave the ward, as they may become very upset. Instead, try accompanying them a little way and then diverting their attention so that you can return to the ward together.

- If a patient does wander off, try not to show anger or anxiety when you do find them. Reassure them and try to get them back into familiar surroundings and a familiar routine as quickly as possible.

- Electronic alarm systems are available that will trigger when a door is opened - this may help if the patient has their own room and is told to remain there. There are also more sophisticated alarm systems that will sound if the patient passes a certain location in the ward.

AND FINALLY ...

To help YOU cope with the stress of dealing with brain injured patients and their families -
- Stay calm
- Take a break
- Talk to others with knowledge and experience of similar problems
- Find out more information from relevant sources (patient organizations, library, the Internet, etc.)
- Refer to this booklet from time to time

Printed in Great Britain
by Amazon